A Long Way to Heaven:

The Caretaker's Tale

Gloria Hanson

2014

A Long Way to Heaven

The Caretaker's Tale

By

Copyright © 2014   Gloria Hanson

ISBN: 1500785946

EAN-13: 9781500785949

Front Cover Art by Richard W. Hanson ©1989

A Note to the Reader

As you read this book, you will notice certain dated entries. These are entries from my blog: https://malatia.wordpress.com

I began writing a blog in 2008 when I realized that friends and family would like to know about my husband's health and treatment. I also came to understand that writing about our experiences helped me, the caregiver, to express my thoughts and feelings in a safe environment, the blogosphere, where the words could be privatized or publicized, read or ignored. The feedback was so positive that this became a welcomed respite for me as I struggled with this new life as a caregiver.

In 2012, I decided to write a very personal blog where I would attempt to express my very private thoughts and feelings regardless of their redeeming or condemning content. Poetry also found its way to this site. This, too, was cathartic and beneficial to my mental health.

You might want to join the blog writing community and reap its benefits.

Gloria Hanson

Chapter 1

Prelude

*"I, Gloria Lucchesi, take you,
Richard Hanson, to be my lawfully
wedded husband, to have and to hold,
from this day forward for better, for
worse, for richer, for poorer, in
sickness and in health, until death do
us part." [Catholic Wedding Vows.
Rite of Marriage, Our Sunday Visitor,
Retrieved 07 June, 2014]*

And that was the beginning of a long and fruitful
relationship between the two oldest children of
immigrants from Italian, Irish and Danish stock.
The road travelled was bumpy, hilly and circuitous
as we ventured many miles. Through many states,
we rode our roller coaster of health, illness and
death–seeking opportunities in career, treatments
and victory over the Grim Reaper and his minion,

the Emperor of All Maladies, cancer.

At first blush, I remember falling in love with Richard in 1959 as he walked bow-legged, clutching his pipe and a copy of Scientific American. He was strolling along Waterman Street as he made his way to the Biology Department at Brown University. Little did I know that the first assault on his rugged body came from a fungal organism called *Tinea cruris*.

The look of discomfort and vulnerability on that handsome face drew me into his world and elicited that caretaking feeling that would become part of my *raison d'être*. There was no escape, and my world began to revolve around him. I had been a selfish, spoiled girl who thought of herself, her ambition, and her career, until lust, love, marriage and children turned me into a circling planet in a sometimes-chaotic universe. We married in June of 1961 and started our family in 1962 since the thinking at the time cautioned against having children after the age of 30. Eggs or sperm of that advanced age might result in severe retardation of children. Richard meanwhile, battled that assault from the invading organisms on his own and controlled the spread of the infection that plagued him for the rest of his life.

His time in the United States Army presented more encounters with the dangers of the living world. Following completion of his Reserve Officers Training Program and a PhD in

Biochemistry, Richard moved his little family of wife and 2 young sons to Colorado. As a second lieutenant assigned to the Army Nutrition Lab at Fitzsimons Hospital in Denver, he did not meet the enemy abroad, rather, he confronted an enemy from the world of viruses. He developed a dangerous case of shingles in the optic nerve of his right eye. As he closed in on potential blindness, he fought to get the only aggressive treatment available in 1963 – massive doses of steroid that stemmed the march of the Herpes zoster virus. He dodged the bullet again and suffered only minor changes in his vision. The family unit was spared a potential threat to their psychological and financial wellbeing.

The next move across the country with 2 kids and our dog, Puli, ended in Conshohocken, Pennsylvania, where we rented a home on Fayette Street. It was a 3-story house with a huge oak tree in the backyard and plenty of room for the rambunctious boys to play and a third floor art room where we could pursue any latent artistic talent any of us might be hiding.

Following the birth of our third child and only daughter in 1966, Richard, who had landed a post-doctoral fellowship in the laboratory of the famous Dr. Sidney Weinhouse, had gone on a trip to Germany for a scientific conference. On a return flight on Lufthansa Airlines, he sat and watched as one of the engines separated from the plane on take-off. He thought that he would be leaving a widow with three young children to fend for themselves in a newly purchased home in Spring Mill, but with the luck of the Irish he made it home safely from his second non-war experience. I describe these assaults and threats in order to lay the groundwork for what is to follow.

The sixties, seventies and eighties rolled by as we settled into our community, made friends, visited family and took care of the business of parenting and career building. While Richard toiled in the laboratory, Gloria worked part-time translating scientific articles, running the household and chasing 3 little ones.

The years of chaos and confusion in society during the Vietnam War, the Civil Rights Movement, the Women's Movement, and the "Don't trust anyone over 30 thinking" spilled over into our family; but we coped as best we could with changing times, adolescent angst and the decline of our parents' health.

Then in 1978 we made the decision to move to Cleveland where Richard would take the job as Chairman of the Biochemistry Department at Case Western Reserve University. The caravan of Ford station wagon carrying 3 very unhappy adolescents, a cowed dog and household plants followed by a smaller Chevy roadster brought us into the mid-west city of Cleveland on a dark June night. More pressure, more stressors took their toll on the somewhat-balanced life we had been living, but we rolled with the punches, worked together to keep our family intact and our marriage on track in a big Tudor-style house on Berkshire Road in Cleveland Heights.

We were in the process of making plans to visit India with some dear friends in September of 1994 when Richard and I were taken by surprise as the ground shook underneath our feet.

Chapter 2

Introduction to the World of the Unwell – the Diagnosis

Chronic Lymphocytic Leukemia was the diagnosis Dr. Adrian Schnall, the internist, gave Richard following routine tests done for the yearly physical on August 8,1994. There was nothing to do at the time since the count was relatively low (15,000 while the norm was 4.5-11 K/uL; white blood cells fight infections and are measured in thousands per cubic millimeter so 4.8 is 4800 cells). There were no signs of troubling symptoms yet so he suggested we go home and watch and wait. That was exactly what we did, setting aside our fears and trepidations. We did watch, carefully, as sometimes cell counts would rise ever so slowly that the person would die of some other malady.

We watched as some family marriages unraveled, our children pursued graduate degrees, four people were convicted in the bombing of the

World Trade Center, O.J. Simpson was arrested in the killings of his wife and her friend, President Clinton was accused of sexual harassment while Governor, and the Supreme Court approved limits on abortion protests. Atrocities in Sarajevo and Rwanda lay to rest the hope for a peaceful world of the future. We listened as Whitney Houston sang our song, 'I Will Always Love You,' and we watched as *Forest Gump* and *Schindler's List* helped us avoid the reality of entering that unknown universe of the unwell.

The 'Watch and Wait' lifestyle was not easy. It is one thing to say it, but it is quite another to be able to set the knowledge aside and live as if nothing had changed. The life of caution, risk avoidance and vigilance had arrived. We unconsciously prepared for war because we feared more attacks. Be prepared, line up your resources, get ready for the worst despite the not knowing; but in the meantime, live life and enjoy. Enjoy yourself, enjoy yourself.

It's Later Than You Think.

Chapter 3

The Dragon Raises Its Ugly Head

Dr. Robert Kellermeyer, the first oncologist to treat Richard, wrote to Dr. Michael Keating, the star researcher at the premier laboratory studying blood cancers, MD Anderson in Houston, Texas:

"On routine physical examination by his primary care physician in 1994, Richard Hanson was found to have an elevated white count to approximately 15,000 with a pre-dominance of lymphocytes. There was no increase in blasts in the bone marrow at this time. His white blood cell count increased slightly through 1996 although his hematocrit and platelet count remained absolutely stable. He then avoided further visits until late 1999 when his white cell count had increased to 41,000 and his weight had dropped to 180 lbs. (13 lbs. from the time of diagnosis)"

In the spring, summer and early fall of 2000 Richard developed an enlarged spleen and generalized lymphadenopathy (palpable enlargement of the lymph nodes), night sweats, anorexia and fatigue followed by prostatitis and difficulty urinating – then came the edema in his right leg and scrotal area. The oncologists agreed: now was the time to respond with treatment. The disease had finally showed its ugly head.

The first chemotherapy was administered on November 29,2000. Fludarabine and cyclophos-phamide (Cytoxan) were the drugs of choice. The former agent suppresses the synthesis of DNA so that the multiplying cells are stopped in their tracks while Fludarabine stops the cells from repairing their DNA. In addition, the antibody, Rituximab was tried, but Richard developed rigors and had a near-death experience. Needless to say, they discontinued that one. Rituximab is a monoclonal antibody that binds to CD 20, present on lymphocytes and is found in patients with B-cell leukemia. The CD20 is a B-lymphocyte antigen on the surface of B cells that enables B-cell immune response. It is the target of Rituximab and useful in the induction of cell death or apoptosis.

What was the result of these 6 treatments? A wonderful six-year remission filled us with relief and joy. In 2000, we moved from our big old, drafty Cleveland Heights home to a light-filled, condominium apartment across from the Rocke-feller Parkland, from a three-story house to a living space on one floor. Sickness had taught us to plan ahead for rainy days. The cloudy future helped us to look ahead to a different reality.

Life was good, we thought. Let's enjoy the time we have together, and so we did. We became grandparents, acquired a son-in-law and spent a sabbatical year at Princeton University. We reconnected with old friends and Richard's New Jersey family, traveled some but stayed close to home, to doctors, to safe places and people. This was the real beginning of a risk management lifestyle. It was difficult to predict the weather and our future. There was no complete remission, no cure, no sure thing, just more watching and waiting.

Chapter 4

2006 and Beyond–
And Now For the Interlude

Dr. Kellermeyer retired and transferred Richard to Dr. Koch who then left the University and brought Dr. Brenda Cooper to take up the mantle of care. Cell counts began rising again, and Fludarabine/Rituximab were the drugs of choice. Infusions were performed more slowly with steroids moderating the effects of the treatment. In 2008, I began to write a blog to inform our friends and family about Richard's health. This Word Press Blog, *https://malatia.wordpress.com* would shield us from well-meaning phone calls and requests for information, and it would serve as an outlet for me to express my thoughts, feelings, and complaints.

The first entry was on January 7, 2008; I wrote, Yes, the disease is progressing – speeding along. The cells are dividing at a faster pace; and the man, my husband of almost 47 years, is becoming more easily fatigued, sweating at night and eating less. He continues to act as if nothing is wrong during the day, but come sundown he hits the wall and needs rest, quiet and sleep. He keeps chugging along, but it comes at a price.

The treatment brought out a new Richard – a steroid-enhanced one who became easily irritated and agitated. This personality change lasted for a week and was followed by the old mellow Richard.

February brought tiredness and calm. He spends his days working at home, talking on the phone, listening to music, watching television and reading. He seems to want to talk about things: work, kids, the new teaching curriculum in the medical school, politics and funeral arrangements.

Well, Richard is in recovery. I know, because he is back to drinking red wine with dinner. A few days into his chemotherapy his stomach could not tolerate much and particularly odious was wine.

He now sleeps better, eats and has a little more energy. He has gained two pounds. He has spread out all over the house – the desk for his art, the dining room table for his Sirius radio, books and journals and his study with a new chair and bookcase. As long as he is happy, he is free to take over the whole house. (2/14/08)

Remission for eight months boosted our spirits as we traveled to Ohio State University to hear that the oncology experts there would not recommend "mopping up" with Campath (Alemtuzumab, a recombinant DNA-derived humanized monoclonal antibody that clears out cancer cells) because of the toxicity. They declared that Richard was in complete remission and should consider clinical trials should his white blood cell count rise.

The beginning of 2009 was calm, but spring brought surprises. In May, Richard developed Toxoplasmosis in his left eye. This infection is caused by Toxoplasma gondii, a protozoa or single celled organism that lives in a parasite and enters the body through infection from a cat or raw meat. It causes posterior uveitis or inflammation in the back of the eye. Treatment resulted in a clearing of the inflammation but required periodic examinations at the Cleveland Clinic since the infection can re-occur.

As if this were not enough, Richard developed a serious bronchitis requiring him to take a strong antibiotic, Levaquin that had been implicated in tendinitis or a tear in the Achilles tendon (tendons are fibrous tissue that connects a bone to a muscle). Ice, stretching, physical therapy, a boot and ibuprofen reduced the inflammation, but it took several months. Meanwhile, Mr. Richard switched from walking to cycling since this sport put less stress on the Achilles tendon. Unfortunately, while riding his bike, he fell and broke the head of his radius (elbow). The chronic bronchitis did not disappear, and lung infections brought him into the care of another specialist, the pulmonologist who gave him antibiotics, an inhaler and a device to loosen the phlegm in his lungs.

"Frustrated Woman"
What is this thing called men?
I wonder what is on the Y chromosome to regulate thinking and judgment. On a Saturday in June 2009, Richard insisted on going on a bike ride with his son and grandson. He had been on a 10-mile trial run the week before, and there was no dissuading him from going on a longer run. Upon my arrival home in the early afternoon, I heard him calling my name in the way he does when something is wrong.

He appears – to show me his wounds – bleeding knee, a long scrape on the opposite leg and a sore arm and shoulder. I took a deep breath; and in my most clinical, unemotional demeanor, I suggested he take ibuprofen and put ice on his sore appendages. On Monday he visited his internist, who told him he had broken the head of his radius and to stay off his bike for 6 weeks. What is wrong with walking? Not macho enough? Something for sissies? Please help me understand before I strangle the poor guy.

The white cell count rose until December when it reached 90,000, and a regimen of Bendamustin (an alkylating agent that works by interfering with DNA duplication) and Rituximab dropped the cells to 59,000. The infusions continued until May 2010 when the cell count came in at 2300. This small triumph came with a price. Richard experienced more frequent lung infections, tiredness, low red blood cell counts, low platelets resulting in nose-bleeds and bruises on his arms that he covered with colorful arm bands. I experienced more frustration and humorless days and nights. He felt embattled and critical of everyone and everything.

I asked him what would make him happy. A train ride was what the man desperately wanted. He had romanticized a trip across the northern United States so here is how it unfolded:

Trip of a Lifetime:
The Empire Builder, an All-American Rail Experience

Leaving Emerald City, the Empire Builder hugs the shores of Puget Sound as it crosses the bridge and marina where threading a needle allows the waters of Salmon Bay and Shilshole Bay to merge. Following the Skykomish River where prospectors and railroad men battled nature years ago when the nation was building. Up 2800 feet we go, gliding along the McKinley highway.

Tall hemlocks, firs and pines reaching – new growth after the clearcut, up from the canyon floor.

Creeks and rivers wind their way through Cascade Mountains capped in snow.

Look down to rushing creeks, lush and light green deciduous plants clinging to the mountain slant.

Look up and watch the snow melt, forming rivulets rushing down to the valley below.

Look sideways and see the sharp-edged rock blasted to make way for us, fallen trees and logs lying by the tracks, nature's pruning making way for new life.

Nearing humankind, watch the dirt roads leading to hidden houses or trailers housing the workers.

Cascade tunnel under Stevens Pass, built in 1929, the longest 7.8 miles by immigrant hands, sweaty and solid stock, full of hope and awe of their adopted country.

Go west, young man, there you'll find gold and wealth.

Human intrusion traverses skyward as wires link settlements, roads lead to logging camps and who knows what.

In Montana the flat lands hold fields of winter wheat on long, harvested and fallow fields against the distant Bear Paw Mountains.

Cottonwoods grow near any available water. Outcroppings, big sky country, fields, broken, rusty vehicles mar the view.

Ranges where one expects to see an Indian Chief and his braves, colorful against the blue sky, looking down on the iron giant passing through the buttes.

In North Dakota oil wells dot the landscape, strewn with pipes, machinery, detritus of that industry, near grasslands with grazing cows, heifers and horses munching grass.

The mighty, muddy Mississippi whose origins lie in the Boundary Waters allows us to see its majestic beauty for 140 miles before making its way south to Louisiana.

The rest of the trip to Chicago is uneventful as we travel the great Midwest with its farmlands and small towns.

Despite the crowded quarters of our unit, the "about to turn" appearance of the train itself, the trip was what was needed by one who had a torn Achilles tendon and a newly acquired lease on life.

Gloria Hanson
June, 2010

Richard can make a silk purse out of a sow's ear. Unfortunately, that gift is not in my genes. I do think, however, that the love affair with the train is over for him – although I am not certain. We'll see, but, if not – he will be flying solo. (May, 2010)

Chapter 5

Ricky Fest and the Letdown

The summer of 2010 flew by ever so peacefully. Richard was able to work as a professor and researcher, and we enjoyed Cleveland in summer. The Emerald Necklace of parks, the Cumberland pool and summer music concerts kept us in good spirits and in hopeful but cautious anticipation.

Richard was relieved because he did not want to be an isolated invalid again and become susceptible to all of the pathogens lurking to attack an immune-compromised individual. I was happy for him and for myself. I wouldn't have to play the guardian at the gate keeping "bugs" at bay – at least for now. Of course, I can continue to be the nagger who pushes food, forbids travel and keeps the husband under lock and key, especially since infections are a risk factor 4-6 months post-treatment. Some job descriptions do change with the recovering economy or the recovering patient.

L'Allegra (The Former Penserosa)

No more guardian at the gate
fending off the germs come late.
I am free to frolic, kick up my heels
while preparing delicious healthy meals.
Come all ye family, friends, gather near.
Let's live it up for another fun-filled year
Gloria's personal blog

In September 2010, the Case Western Reserve University Medical School administration and faculty, with the financial backing of other institutions and friends, planned a celebration for Richard's contributions as professor and good citizen of this Cleveland academic institution. A full-day event, this symposium and an elaborate dinner and program devoted to praising this dear husband of mine were such a joy for Richard. Not only were his colleagues and former students in attendance, but the party also included members of my family and Richard's. It was an immense success, although his little woman could see that it was wearing on him. However, he rose to the occasion and became his charming, ebullient mayoral self with platelets at a healthy 64,000.

Later in the fall of 2010, the party was over. The cell count began to rise again. Dr. Cooper referred Richard to OSU where treatment with Flavopiridol and Lenalinimide was being evaluated. The former is a synthetic flavonoid based on an extract from an Indian plant. It works by inhibiting certain kinases thereby arresting cell division and causing apoptosis. Lenalinimide is a derivative of thalidomide and induces apoptosis.

On October 20, 2010 Richard and I travelled to Columbus, Ohio to visit Dr. Michael Grever at Ohio State James Cancer Center. Dr. Grever reviewed the treatment records and described his research on the drug, Flavopiridol, an agent that is effective against p53-mutated chronic lymphocytic leukemia. He and his colleagues were conducting a phase 1 clinical trial of Flavopiridol and Lenalinimide to attack these highly resistant mutated cells.

There it was – an entry into the world of clinical trials because the standard regular toolbox was empty. Clinical trials are studies designed to test new drugs or combinations of drugs, as well as evaluate diagnostic, preventive and treatment methods. In 3 phases, the team of doctors, nurses and researchers work to determine how and whether the drug or treatment works; at what dosage the drug is effective and how safe it is for patients. Since this is an experimental approach, there are no guarantees. Only after the experimental drug or procedure passes all three stages, is it eligible to be considered for approval by the Federal Drug Agency.

This is a new ballgame since the suggested regimen for Richard includes a 3-week series of 2-3 day hospitalizations where the drugs are administered intravenously. This is followed by a 2-week respite, and then the cycle is repeated 2 more times with the hope of a one-year remission. The language has changed, the assaults have become more virulent, and the fight team now includes a kind of "Navy Seal" group who specialize in the aggressive battles against those quickly moving cells that have increased in numbers and have challenged the patient and his doctors to a battle until the end.

We drove to Columbus on November 3 and traveled to the James Cancer Center to begin the process: a 10-hour hydration and surgery to install a mediport into the left subclavian vein, inserting a plastic object with 2 ports where they could administer drugs without having to "stick" him every time they had to take blood or infuse drugs. The next morning the competent and friendly oncology nurses began the 4-hour Flavopiridol infusion of Cycle 1 week 1.

Many tubes and many draws to check uric acid, cystine and potassium levels insured that he did not have tumor lysis syndrome (a metabolic condition resulting from the breakdown of products from dying cancer cells that can result in acute renal failure). The discharge on Saturday by the nurse practitioner who called him the 'perfect professor' because of his response to treatment (white cell count dropped to 33,000 from 69,000), his good blood work and his friendly, energetic attitude – and certainly not to ignore his handsome gentleman's hat kept nearby.

Cycle 1, week 2 went well. No major side effects, although the steroids turned him into a chatty fella, albeit a little hyper-chatty fella. He is basically a 'Most Happy Fella' so I can deal with that. The underlying stress of this process follows me as we drive to Cleveland. I surrender to my weary bones and get a good night's sleep. Having Richard safe in our bubble-mattress bed re-assures me that everything will be okay – at least for today. Tomorrow I will be ready for my cardio-muscle class that helps to relieve the pressure. Sweat and beating heart work wonders, feeding my resolve and giving me strength.

Cycle 1, week 3 is now complete. Steroids are wearing off. There is, no chattiness, but he is still working at his computer. He feels a little tired but tells me he is okay. Tomorrow he sees Dr. Cooper here in Cleveland and receives more steroids and a Neulasta shot (At $7000. per!) His neutrophils (a type of white blood cells that fight infections) are down, so this medication should give him a boost.

One wonders what happens to the poor souls without health insurance or on Medicaid. Would they be able to get such an expensive medication? Or how about those patients in rural America who do not get treated at a state of the art medical center – what happens to them? Okay, enough politics and existential angst. We will return to Columbus on December 6 for the next round, and, hopefully there will be a little global warming so we don't have to drive on icy or snowy roads. *(Nov. 2, 2010)*

In December Richard started on Cycle 2 week 1, with the addition of Lenalinimide that "flushed out" cells in the lymph nodes and bone marrow, transporting those mutated B cells to the blood for destruction and thereby resulting in an elevation of the blood cell count. Initially we were surprised that the cell count had risen; but Dr. John Byrd, Dr. Grever's associate, who was now in charge of Richard's care, assured us that this was a common "flush." In Cycle 2, week 2 the white blood cell count went from 33,000 to 18,000. Hopefully that is sustainable for longer than a few months.

We were both happy to be home on Friday. Richard then dropped off the 'old bag' plus the travel bags, and rushed down to the Biochemistry Department to attend the Christmas party and sing a few old songs. Steroids really do give the guy a boost. *(December, 2010)*

The new year of 2011 was bound to be better than the last twelve months, we hoped. It did not start off that way. When we arrived in Columbus we were told that Richard's neutrophil count was too low to continue with week 2 of Cycle 2. We called for a draft of all eligible neutrophils that were willing to fight for their owner.

This time of the Egyptian Arab Spring revolution had put us in a military state of mind. We were ready to continue the long trips to Columbus, the bed bug capital that year, to continue the struggle if the OSU team could try to re-commence the treatment.

On January 26, we got our wish for continued treatment but were shocked to hear that the mutated B cells had lost all common sense and instead of going down in number were heading up – 80-100,000. Dr. Byrd and Dr. Grever did not understand why this was happening since Richard did not have "bulky" disease where the mutated cells crowd out the healthy red and white cells or deposit in the lymph nodes. This was a phase 1 clinical trial for this combination of drugs and was designed to discover proper dosages for this medication.

The doctors told us to return for week 2 of Cycle 3 next week, and then they would determine whether this regimen would continue or whether they would switch to another clinical trial with another drug. I had just received my infusion– hope, and we happily drove home to our light-filled condo and to all things familiar. On February 4, following an examination of the results of the morning blood work, Doctors Grever and Byrd delivered their verdict. The Flavopiridol and Lenalinimide cocktail was not working well enough to continue.

Go home and get that platelet count up to over 100,000 and return for a new combination we have in mind. This is the long and short of it: the big fight has been delayed. The generals are planning their next attack, and we have gone back to our bunkers for reflection and restoration. Meanwhile, this mini platoon will be in training–a little exercise, good food and reasonable isolation. No infections are allowed to travel to those bronchiectic lungs, especially with all the sanitizing wipes and masks in every corner.

'You think the Egyptian people are fighters – you ain't seen nuttin' yet.'

Chapter 6

Another Trial, Another Wait–
The PCI Drone Adventure

March 3, 2011 – a trip to headquarters is planned to coordinate strategy to fight those mutated cells that were on the march as the platelet corps was in decline. Here is the attack plan: a Phase 1 trial of a Bruton tyrosine kinase inhibitor together with the monoclonal antibody Ofatumumab would hopefully increase cell death or apoptosis. Since Richard does not have the P53 gene on Chromosome 17, his mutated cells don't die off normally. As a result the mutated cells are dividing and accumulating in the blood and crowding out the healthy cells. Those clones will do anything to stay alive and replicate. He can join this trial in 4 weeks, and meanwhile Richard will attempt to avoid infections while I will continue to remind, nag and keep him away from any nasty bacteria, viruses or fungi that may attempt to invade. Oh I forgot: control and manipulate are also on my list of duties.

The honeymoon is over. We have been on a holiday of sorts since March 5, 2011;and despite a few rough spots, we managed to avoid major damaging infections or marital battles. Compliance is not a major word in Richard's vocabulary, but he is improving. It must be difficult to give up control to doctors, medications, wife, physician daughter and chronic lymphocytic leukemia.

Tomorrow, April 23, we will travel to Columbus and begin treatment with Bruton tyrosine kinase inhibitor, called PCI-32765 or Ibrutinib, a blocker of B-cell activation and hopefully a signal to the mutated cells that their time is up and they should die. If this drug works then we will return every week for 4 cycles of 2 days per week of treatment together with a monoclonal antibody designed to kick a—and result in remission. Then for cycles 5-8 we will go for a once a month treatment. *(April 22, 2011)*

A week of PCI-32765 has resulted in a lowered total white cell count (154,000 to 127,000) – high but headed in the right direction. Our new Ford Fusion hybrid purchased in January of 2010 has logged 7,000 miles. I have also logged 7,000, but the car looks better than I do. Three weeks later the cells had dropped 30%. There were few side effects. May 27 showed another reduction in the white blood cell count to 86,000.

On June 28 we noted that they have been whacked *Sopranos* style. There is good news from North Park tonight. The total lymphocytes (5,000 bad and 22,000 becoming bad) have decreased to 27,000. They are probably floating somewhere in the East River near the Bada Bing Club. It appears that the combination of PCI (Tony) and Ofatumumab (Paulie Walnuts) whacked them good. More will be whacked on July 4.

Another 4 weeks of treatment will end our weekly trips. Following a short vacation from chemotherapy, we will resume the treatment with monthly visits until January 2012 when this phase of the clinical trial ends. Then we travel into the unknown.

July, August, September, October, November, December of 2011 and January through July of 2012 were months of relative calm as the mutated B cells had met their match and were being beaten back. This was no peace treaty. We knew that, but the 18 months gave Richard a chance to return to some normalcy.

He was the poster boy for PCI, and he began to polish his Beau Brummell reputation when he went to the James Hospital wearing his suit, open collar shirt and the gentlemen's hat. Richard's white blood cell count was in the normal range, but Dr. Byrd would not vouch for any other signs of normalcy in his patient. We will continue to keep our guard up and do the risk/benefit analysis of our every move.

Following a trip to Captiva Island in March where we both spent most of our vacation time in bed with some kind of flu bug that Richard had kindly shared with me, and which laid us both low, we returned to Columbus, only to discover that Richard's cells had increased from 9,000 to 11,000. Those little buggers had been slowly increasing, and now they had finally pushed through the normal range.

"Perhaps this Ibrutinib drug has stopped working on me. Perhaps I need a larger dose," Dr. Hanson surmised as he tried to transform a PhD into an MD.

"No," interrupted Nurse Gloria (trying to transform a Masters in Social Work into a medical degree). "I would suspect that if the drug was not working, it would have become inert and your cell count would be much higher."

Back and forth we went, forward and back as couples do until Richard fell asleep while Gloria had some peace and quiet to drive home on Route 71. A few times, she thought that worrying about death by cancer was futile since we would surely die in a head-on crash with a semi full of widgets for Walmart, or an SUV driven by some high-on-meth addict being chased by the State troopers."

(April, 2011)

In June and July, the enemy had picked up new

recruits. Following surgery for a meniscal tear in his knee and a bout with a Baker's cyst, Richard was ready to "buy the farm." Dr. Byrd advised Richard to stay on the Ibrutinib since he does not have any overt signs of the disease such as enlarged spleen or lymph nodes, night sweats or extreme tiredness. Perhaps there was another kinase operation to slow down cell multiplication and increase apoptosis.

Richard was not convinced and kept telling me to prepare to live alone in the 2800+ square foot condominium. Could I take care of it alone? Make plans, he advised me. Me! The devoted planner (of the 'better to make a plan and then change it than to have no plan at all' philosophy), I responded that I already had begun working on a five-year plan and was currently updating my dating profile. He chuckled but persisted in his glumness. *(July, 2011)*

August 15 brought more bad news in that Richard's cell count had increased by 50,000 in one month. We were in shock and dismayed, even despairing until Dr. Byrd ignited a little flame of hope. He reported that a lab was analyzing Richard's mutated cells and would do a gene sequencing to determine if there was another mutation resulting in a group of resistant cells bypassing the Ibrutinib and using another kinase pathway downstream to avoid death. The doctors should have a plan next month. There was no joy in Mudville that night, but – the mighty Richard had not struck out.

In September, 2011 we received more disheartening news – the white blood cell count increased 97,000 in one month to 200,000. Those terrorist cells found another pathway to survive despite the targeted cell therapy. Two days later Richard received 300 ml of Ofatumumab, a monoclonal antibody, that attacks a broad spectrum of cells – a plan to repeat the infusion 3 more times. This should give him more time on Planet Earth and a chance for a new strategy involving 2 new targeted cell therapies (ABT-199 and GA101).

From Gloria's Personal Blog

Is Life Worth Living?
Darkness is everywhere.
Death lurks in the corners.
We search for distractions
to keep us sane and safe.

Denial of death, I say,
loving, hating, exercising,
conversing, praying–
it is all to no avail.
That existential angst
is still there, following,
swallowing, engulfing,
even in our dreams.

'Enjoy yourself, it's later than you think
Enjoy yourself, while you're still in the pink.
The years go by, as quickly as a wink.
Enjoy yourself. Enjoy yourself.
It's later than you think.'

Music by Carl Sigman, lyrics by Herb Magidson,
1949

Chapter 7

The Lost Week

I am sure you have heard of the award-winning film, *The Lost Weekend* with Ray Milland, especially if you are more than 60 years of age. Well, Richard and I had a 'lost week' in Columbus. We traveled there on September 19 to be bright and early for our treatment meeting with Dr. John Byrd. Following the blood draw and a description of Richard's symptoms (chest pain, trouble urinating, extreme fatigue), we learned that his white cell count was 420,000, up by 100,000 from the previous week.

Immediately, Dr. Byrd told us that he wanted to admit Richard to the hospital and begin a heavy, deep and serious treatment. Initially, following hydration and hydroxy urea infusion, Richard had a CT/PET scan, an Echocardiogram in order to begin the process of blocking DNA replication and to determine the status of his heart.

On Thursday night, my sweet husband underwent a process called leucophoresis whereby blood was removed through a line in the neck's jugular vein, separated by a centrifuge-like machine to remove the white blood cells and then returned to his circulatory system. The first treatment resulted in a drop of the white blood cell count to 285,000, and the second leucophoresis dropped those mutated monsters to 218,000.

On Friday night, Richard started on a new, well-tested regimen, EPOCH-R, a combination therapy of a 'cocktail' of etoposide, doxorubicin and vincristine, followed by a three-minute infusion of cyclophosphamide and a longer treatment with the antibody Rituximab. He tolerated this well, having been saturated with steroids and saline.

This treatment continued until Wednesday at 2PM. He was still Mr. Chatty when they wheeled him down to the Ross Heart Center where the surgeons snipped a port line that was too long and 'tickling' his heart. Full of holes but with an intrepid spirit, he returned to 'his' room 759, in the James Cancer Hospital where he enjoyed a restful sleep with a little help from his friend, Ambien.

Friday was a difficult day for us, and we were so happy that our physician daughter, Daria, flew down from Portland, Maine to be with us. We all, including the patient, were fearful that this was the beginning of the end; however, Dr. Byrd and the wonderful staff of nurses and doctors gave us hope and a difficult but damned effective treatment regimen to bring down those nasties to 37,000. No, it isn't normal –yet, but we have left the depths of despair and are preparing to fight on.

It was a long week, but a worthwhile one both physiologically and emotionally. Facing the Grim Reaper, Richard took his inventory and examined his life, both strengths and weaknesses. He and I also received strong support from our sons and family who rallied around us together with dear friends. Thursday, September 27, we hurried home to Cleveland Heights and sighed, 'Home, Sweet, Home."

Now for those of you who have not dozed off during this long entry, here is my little poem written while I sat watching 'the paint dry'. STOP HERE IF YOU HAVE HAD ENOUGH. I will never know.

Note to the Almighty!

Stanza 1
Alpha and Omega, Jesus, Yahweh, Allah, hear my call!
All you masters of the Universe,

Buddha, Jehovah, Brahma, Great Spirit, Hear my prayers!
Listen to my cries!

Stanza 2
There is a war going on here.
The Emperor of All Maladies
has taken over our lives.
Imperial cells multiply and attack,
leaving nothing in their path,
fighting to squeeze others out, survive.

Stanza 3
The Host Army mobilizes, calls to arms,
responding with vigor as
chemical cocktails fly,
adjunctive antibodies join the fray,
as the noble defense seeks victory.

Stanza 4
The Emperor is stunned and shaken.
The Army sends in re-enforcements
to bring on a surge, a scourge.
Top Brass order a target shooter
to strike, cut off supplies, sever.

Stanza 5
Good, but not enough to end it.
The Emperor will find a way
as cell counts rise swiftly.
The Army reacts, sends big guns,
cutting off supply routs
killing many big B's and little b's.

Stanza 6
The cells fall in droves,
drowning in a bloody path,
looking for escape, safety.
Centurions want to finish them off

Sending EPOCH forces in to the fight,
legionnaires, supernumerarii,
pedites to clean the mess as collateral
damage mounts.

Stanza 7
Is this the endgame, the final battle?
Is true Armageddon near?
Weakened, unbowed,
the Dark Knight rises.
He is ready for another round.
The defeated Emperor is in retreat.
Long live the Valiant Gladiator!

(Gloria Hanson)

Chapter 8

A Little of Everything

October, 2012 brought mixed blessings.
Following the September hospitalization and tough
treatments a subdued Richard came home. He
stayed around the condo, working on his computer
and avoiding human contact with most family and
friends because he understood that the drugs had
seriously compromised his blood profile. Dr.
Cooper and Staff at the Seidman Cancer Center in
Cleveland treated him with Neulasta, platelets and
red blood cells resulting in an improved blood
picture and a revitalized Richard.

We were then ready to travel to Columbus to
see what the generals at OSU had up their sleeves.
Before Richard could enter a new clinical trial of a
promising new drug, ABT199 and a strong
antibody GA101, he would have to have a bridge
therapy with oral AR42 (a histone deacetylase
inhibitor that disrupts DNA replication) to reduce

the number of B cells. Then he would be eligible for the ABT199 drug that had been found to be helpful with refractory CLL, especially for the type that was found mainly in the bone marrow and not in the lymph nodes.   Again, we had to remain in Columbus so that the drug effects could be monitored daily.

Our new little home away from home was the University Inn, an about-to-turn Hotel near the Olentangy River. It was a short distance from the James Cancer Hospital, and we fit right in as we are ripened fruit on the vine. Restaurants, a movie theater, and a Vietnamese manicure salon allowed us to stop and enjoy a little bit of Americana before settling in to Room 117 to watch the news programs that would certainly add to the gloom and doom of the evening if not for the thought that others around the planet lived in more difficult situations than ours – a paradoxical way to lift one's mood.

AR42 worked for a while, and then it didn't.

Richard's white cell count had resumed its rapid multiplication and accumulation during the drug free 9-day hiatus. Dr. Byrd wanted to stop this progression as soon as possible so he planned to hospitalize Richard and treat him with Cyclophosphamide, Rituxan and high dosage steroids for 4-5 days.

One enters the huge OSU Medical Center through an adjacent parking lot, an elevator ride to

Floor 2 where automatic doors usher one into the hospital proper. Walking through the sunlit atrium on polished marble floors one then hikes through well-lit hallways exhibiting non-offensive art and multiple signs leading you to the various departments. Waiting for the slow elevator to the James Cancer hospital floors gives the visitor a chance to wipe off germ-y hands with sanitizer. There are no body sanitizers or face masks yet, but there probably should be given the number of humans in various sizes, states of health and hair quantity coming and going.

On Friday, November 23, Richard traveled to the eighth floor with his rolling computer bag containing copies of *The New Yorker*, a new Barbara Kingsolver novel and his own lab research results from Case Western Reserve University on his computer. He was led to his private room where they would begin his steroid prep before the chemotherapy. With 160mg of Dexamethasone and who knows how much of the other stuff, Richard's body demonstrated amazing abilities to wage war on those mutated B cells and survive. Four days later his cell count was down to 7000 from 271,000.

Hospitals have their own time tables, rhythms and culture, and although we were eager to return home, we had to "cool our jets" until Dr. Jeffrey Jones and his young residents examined Richard, gave him his marching orders and discharged him.

The upbeat staff of nurses and assistants helped him get ready and told him that despite his winsome personality they did not want to see him again soon.

The feeling was mutual as I looked at my husband's handsome face, not believing that he was and is still ill. Our new plan involves a shot of Neulasta to build up his neutrohils so he won't be so vulnerable to infection, transfusions if his platelets are low and weekly Rituxan treatment. This will prepare Richard the Lion-Hearted to be ready for the next battle. *(December, 2012)*

I am tired!
Tired of this roller coaster
ride of waning life,
tired of uncertainty,
the mood swings,
mounting cell counts,
waiting for results
avoiding the crowd.

I am weary of the trips,
of the snail-like strolls,
of loveless nights,
the soft silences,
the sandwiched suppers.

I am fearful of clouds
of sleepless nights,
soul searing days,
sanguine stories,
sotted simplicities.

I am hopeful for now,
For peaceful days,
Panic-free nights,
Purposeful words.
Pensive prayers.

Gloria Hanson

Chapter 9

The End of a Brutal Year

This past year has been a difficult one for Richard as he continues to serve as a research subject for the oncologists at the James and Seidman Cancer Centers. My little guinea pig has continued to respond and survive, but these treatments do take their toll on him as they stem the tide until the aggressive clones work their way around the drugs. The positive attitude is because, in spite of the difficulties, these clinical trials have kept him alive.

Friends and family ask me how I am 'holding up.' With my philosophy of one day at a time, daily exercise, and an innate love of solitude and schedule, I am living this 'new normal' life and feel content to be here. Each day I add a tincture of hope to my morning coffee and move on to meet the day's challenge. I used to plan weeks and months and years ahead, but now I plan for today, tomorrow and maybe next week. Of course this bumpy ride makes me dizzy sometimes, but strangely enough, it has its own pattern and predictability. I am learning how to sit back and enjoy or at least tolerate the ride, and when Richard is on his steroid loquacious rant, I imagine that he is following me around with his banjo. I can dissociate and know that this, too, shall pass.

Richard will continue to receive treatment at the Seidman Cancer Center where he is infused with steroids and the monoclonal antibody, Rituximab. The trial he was waiting for was cancelled as two people died. Do you have a new bag of tricks, Dr. Byrd?

I keep hoping for a John Hanson miracle. John, Richard's father was diagnosed with liver cancer. He was in his early nineties, and the physician told us, following a scan and blood work showing a high level of alpha fetal protein indicating liver disease, that John had about 6 months to live. Tests were repeated, and the results remained the same. Six months came and went, and John was still kicking. The tumors had disappeared, and the doctor could not explain why–either the tests were wrong the first **and** second time or 'this was a miracle.'

However, John Byrd does have a new tool. It is TG-02, an inhibitor of cyclin-dependent kinases and the mutation JAK2 and ERK5 that can interfere with apoptosis. That is what we want–death to that army of mutated B cancer cells. The genetic analysis indicated that Richard has a mutation that interferes with the expression of protein kinas C (PKC) – beta 11 and the activation of the NF-kB signaling pathway in the microenvironment resulting in the survival of the malignant B cells. These little bastard terrorists do not die.

A pain in Richard's right eye and back led to double vision and a few more "sticks" to his lumbar region, an MRI and a neurological workup. The diagnosis was an ischemia in the third cranial nerve that controls eye coordination and stenoses in cervical vertebra 4 and 5, and to top it off, CLL cells in his cerebrospinal fluid. The result of this "million dollar" workup – no clinical trial with TG-02, but yes for infusions of Depocyte or Cytarabine that will get rid of the cells in the spinal fluid.

For now, Richard will receive an infusion of Carfilzomib, a proteosomal inhibitor that is being tested on refractory CLL patients. Since these active B cells produce a lot of protein that is usually degraded by the action of proteosomes, otherwise known as 'little garbage trucks' in the cells. Carfilzomib stops these garbage trucks allowing for the proteins to accumulate in the cells and become targets for the drug to kill. We are now back on the treadmill with drone-like drugs designed to attack the bad 'guys.' Hopefully the collateral damage will be minimal.

That 77-year old body is something else! Gone is the double vision and back pain and down went the CLL cells in the spinal fluid. The other blood work is good so he can come out of the isolation room. To celebrate the 15,000 B cell number, we splurged and ate yummy food at a restaurant in Columbus. We might as well travel wherever on a full stomach. Then we returned to Cleveland to celebrate Easter with our Cleveland family, have another good meal at Giovanni's Italian restaurant with dear friends, attend a Persian wedding ceremony and travel to Costco's to buy blueberries for our morning cereal. Eat, live and be merry!

Richard continued to receive the Carfilzomib and the Depocyte and the results were good. The white blood cell count fell to 8000 in the first week of April, and the cerebrospinal fluid cell count also fell.

My 77th birthday was spent in a hospital room awaiting the nurses who will infuse Richard with Carfilzomib and red blood cells to give him a little energy. I am toying with the idea of going to the movies to see the film about Jackie Robinson, the Negro baseball player who overcame racism to play with the Brooklyn Dodgers. I think I will return and pick Richard up in time for dinner since the day will end at 6:30PM. I don't feel guilty doing this because the plastic chairs are hard and uncomfortable, and he is in good hands. I also have my 'dumb' flip-phone in case something happens.

I have been in a bad mood the last week following the treatment because of an old complaint. Despite the slow recovery from the flu and a hacking cough Richard insisted on going to meetings devoted to the planning for a celebration for Julian Stanczack, a noted Cleveland artist. In bed before the meetings and in bed after the meetings, he cancelled a dinner and concert invitation from his friend and stayed home. I attended and again felt no guilt.

On Saturday afternoon he insisted on going to a baseball game and sitting outside the loge on a cold, rainy day. Of course he came home with a bad cough and a deadening fatigue. Bed, bed and more bed, and I feel disheartened when he does not take care of himself. I realize that I can't want more for him than he wants for himself, but I also see that I am at the end of the line as he uses his available energy at work or work related events. This is not anything new, but earlier in our marriage I had the freedom to go where I wanted, travel and be independent. Now my life is constricted. I sit around waiting for the next trip to Columbus, the next taxi service ride to work or hospital. If he took better care of himself, I would not mind the caretaking duty, but the poor judgment calls leave me breathless and fighting resentment.

Gloria's Personal Blog

Dr. Cooper wondered whether Richard might benefit from a shunt placed in his skull and a new drug, Methotrexate that would kill off the remaining CLL cells. Dr. Byrd on the other hand, has arranged a meeting with Dr. David Porter who has been developing A CAR 1 treatment where T cells are removed from the patient's blood, re-engineered to destroy the mutated B cells and then re-introduced into the patient's blood stream using a viral vector. These changed fighters then go to work to destroy the CLL terrorists. It could be a great final battle victory if it worked. The schedule is daunting–6-8 weeks in hospital area so they can respond to any serious cytokine or other allergic reaction. Our trip to Philadelphia ended with the pronouncement by this Wizard of Oz that T-cell treatment was out of the question for now because Richard would have to be free of any CLL cells in his spinal fluid.

Relieved? Yes, we were both conflicted, but also relieved because neither one of us were so enthusiastic about this treatment for a 77 year-old. I must admit to also being relieved that I would not have to leave my home, my tennis and my gym buddies and other friends and family for 6-8 weeks. I know those are selfish reasons, but they were secondary to my fears that I would lose my husband in a catastrophic cytokine storm. I am not ready to let him go yet. Not only can he drive at night, but also he can open jars. We celebrated with a delicious meal at a Chinese fusion restaurant. So the trip on the yellow brick road did not end badly after all. There seems to be a silver lining in these trips to the land of the unwell in pursuit of life, and we manage to find joy and peace in there somewhere – food, friends, family.

Following a 2-week "vacation" from Columbus we returned for a final lumbar injection for his leptomeningeal metastasis (this was the first time I recall this term being used) and a suggestion from Dr. Byrd that we wait a month or 2 to re-evaluate the cells metastisized into the spinal fluid. There would be no hole bored into hubby's skull. I cannot count the number of holes or injections made into my honey's sagging skin by well-meaning nurses, residents, and doctors. At the very least they should follow up with a little Botox. Perhaps I could get in line, too, should they decide to call in another specialist – the dermatologist. Dr. Byrd sprinkled more fairy dust on us as he described his 2 new possibilities if Carfilzomib stops working: ABT199 and IP1145.

I love that guy in spite of the fact that he sent us on a wild goose chase to Philadelphia to see the Wizard. Of course, nothing much was said about

that trip. Richard put a positive spin on the trip –
a greater understanding of the science, the treatment and the side effects. I, on the other hand,
would have questioned the reasoning behind
sending Richard on this long trip given the novelty
of the procedure and the reported scary side
effects. This is why Richard will have to wait for me
while I do my purgatorial time while he is up in
heaven having tea with Mother Teresa.

Chapter 10

A New Direction

The latter part of June, 2013 brought a new set of problems – cramps and pain in the thighs, and later, chills, shaking and vomiting following the infusions of the Carfilzomib. The second treatment the following day brought warm tingling feeling in the thighs as the pain intensified. There had been no addition of steroid to the regimen for almost a week, and since he could not sleep at night, he thought he might see if the addition of a steroid tablet could quell the pain. Voilà, the pain was gone! Richard "House" had tested his hypothesis, and for the moment the results confirmed his idea. Team Byrd did not buy it.

Dr. Byrd then discontinued the Carfilzomib because he thought that that the ataxia and muscle cramps may have been caused by the drug. He also surmised that the CLL cells in the spinal fluid might have been implicated and ordered a lumbar tap and an MRI of the brain to check whether the cells had migrated to his brain causing the reported symptoms. He also suggested a new approach – the infusion of a systemic chemotherapy drug, Cladribine that crosses the blood/brain barrier. The downside included an increased susceptibility to infection. Luckily my helicopter wife license had not expired, and we would settle down in our air-conditioned condo with our books and the remaining episodes of "Breaking Bad," realizing that life can be beautiful for us, but not for Walter and Jesse.

The Cladribine infusions performed in Cleveland in July and August were successful in reducing the number of mutated B cells in his spinal fluid to 54, slowly replicating types that could be controlled with subsequent treatments of Cladribine and Rituximab. If the cell count fell to 5 or below, Richard would be eligible to return to a targeted cell therapy. This little respite from Columbus was a welcome relief for us, but the news that members of our family and several of our friends were struggling with cancer did not make for a peaceful summer.

This whole business of dying in a medical-ized way has me doubting the whole process. If one has a late stage cancer diagnosed, why would one want to struggle for a few months of life? Being poked, radiated, cut and drugged

in order to breathe a few more breaths?
My experiences in the past with this
turtle's race to death has turned me
away from trying to prolong life if it is
futile. I can understand wanting to help by
participating in clinical trials, but if the
prognosis is dire, give in and embrace
your end. Start rehearsing for your role
despite the chance that you might forget
the dialogue once you are faced with the
Grim Reaper. Challenge your negative
thinking about death and concentrate
on the benefits of dying well. Be prepared
to become part of the universe, to hopefully join your relatives and friends in
the spiritual mass of humanity, to con-
tribute your atoms to the renewal of life."

Gloria's Personal Blog

Despite the benefits of the Cladribine treatment on his spinal fluid cancer cells, Richard has
developed ataxia where his gait is compromised,
and his balance is off. He also takes a long time
with buttons, getting dressed and walking from
one place to another. His hearing is compromised,
as well, and warts have grown on his fingers. He is
discouraged and despairing, but he goes on with
his work and his life. He finds that walking helps to
improve his gait and his mood. He dons his walking

shoes, bright green shirt, jacket, hat, arm pro-
tectors, iPod and cane (one of many as you would
suspect from this habitual collector of things) and
cuts quite a figure in the early morning light as he
walks to the track near our home and goes round
and round for 3 to 4 miles. A positive attitude
makes a difference when one faces adversity. That
sounds banal, but I have come to believe this as I
watch my wobbly warrior.

We were missing our trips to Columbus so we
decided to take a ride to pay a visit to the oncologist, John Byrd. After all, he is the main man in
this battle of the cells. The main woman, Dr.
Brenda Cooper, takes care of treatment here in
Cleveland. They are the quarterbacks for a team of
doctors taking care of different ailing body parts of
Richard Winfield Hanson, 77, who is still kicking by
maintaining for the last 10 months that he is 78.
His birthday is around the corner on November 10
at which time he will actually be 78 and not play
rounding up. The team, actually more like a
battalion, includes a dermatologist, ophthalmol-
ogist, internist, dentist, infectious disease specialist, pulmonologist, ear, nose and throat doctor,
orthopedist, urologist, physical therapist, neurologist, hospitalist and oncologists. We could add a
psychologist, but we won't go there.

(October, 2013)

Dr. Byrd advised Richard to continue with 2 more rounds of Cladribine because this systemic drug is keeping his cancer cells in check, pursue physical therapy for the cervical stenosis and ataxia while the neurologist in Cleveland examines all of his medical records from the James and Seidman Centers and then consults with the Generals for a diagnosis and treatment plan for these new symptoms. (November, 2013)

Guess what? That examination and consultation never happened. We will never know why, but we have our hypotheses. We certainly don't want to think that part of that team has given up on the old guy because of his neurological symptoms.

The 2 harpies, wife and daughter, ganged up on poor Richard telling him that perhaps the ataxia that is resulting in more buckled legs and falls might be due to the Ambien and Ativan he has been taking for sleep. However, until his doctor friend made the same suggestion during a telephone conversation, he would not change his mind. I could become resentful and negative, but I need all the help I can get to insure compliance since a fall and broken hip would put him and me in an even worse place – a drop to another level. That is why I can't stop the encouragement, the hovering, nagging (?) and so on and on and on.

Chapter 11

What a Difference a Day Makes

Life is full of little surprises. On November 7, 2013, Richard complained of a pain on the front of his right leg. He insisted on going to work but asked me to pick him up in the early afternoon. He went to bed as soon as we arrived home. 'A good nap will cure the pain.' Two hours later he woke with the shakes, chills and a fever of 101.6 F. He showed me his leg. I was aghast! The shin was now a reddish-purple color, warm to the touch and sensitive. In my most loving nurse/wife voice I suggested we go to the emergency room.

"Certainly not!"

I recognized that Richard – noncompliant, stubborn-as-his Dad voice and left the room to call his oncologist who told me to take him to the Emergency Room immediately. Returning to face the ogre, I relayed Dr. Cooper's message. She had alerted the staff to his arrival.

"Okay, okay." Grumble, grumble.

Off we went, and lucky that we did. The doctors found Escheridia coli in his blood and admitted him to the Seidman Cancer Center at 4AM in the morning and started him on a specific penicillin-like antibiotic. The infectious disease team took over the hovering and lecturing, telling him that any sign of fever or infection should point him to the ER. Listen to your wife, they wisely counseled. One of the woman doctors with a wonderful sense of humor said that good judgment is an X-related trait, and women have 2 X's while men have only 1. There is no scientific evidence to prove this hypothesis, but there certainly is plenty of anecdotal data.

On November 10, the lucky patient's birthday, the infectious disease team (doctors, nurses, aides, residents, medical students) at this teaching hospital bid him farewell, sending him home with CefTRIAXone antiobiotic to be infused at home by team Hanson (Gloria and Richard) following the instructions of the home health care nurse. The patient, a subdued version of the guy who went in 3 days ago promises to stay home for the remainder of the treatment schedule and work from home. Let's see if he "walks the talk."

During our nightly fireside chats, Richard came up with a new theme. He wants me to go out and find another

man with whom I could have an affair
since he – my husband – has ruined
my life. He is convinced of it and thinks
I am too kind to tell him the truth. I tell
him that by no means has he 'ruined
my life' since I live for the most part as I
would live without him. He does not
believe that I don't want to travel or go
out and about. He becomes very emo-
tional, and I listen, comfort him and
try to re-assure him that my life is good,
having him around, and that caring for
him is what I want for this moment in
time.

When nothing seems to work, I
retreat into humor and tell him that I will
give this some thought before I pick out
my "victim" and try to fit him into my
busy schedule, keeping him waiting until
I tuck Richard in for the night and then
the new boyfriend and I can 'party'–at
least until 10PM."

Gloria's Personal Blog

Chapter 12

More Bumps in the Road

The end of the year has arrived, and we were hoping for stable times and a bug-free Richard since his infected, reddish-purple leg is now a "pasty" white matching his left leg and body. The Lone Ranger has dodged another bullet; however, the neurological symptoms persist and have increased as he has weakness in his legs, loss of sensation in his fingertips and toes and a very unsteady gait. We still have no clue as to the cause. The doctors agree that the Cladribine is lowering the mutated B cells in the spinal fluid, but it is also killing important blood cells such as platelets and red blood cells. This is not good. Richard has decided to put off his sky diving lessons with the low numbers of oxygen-rich cells. They plan another lumbar puncture in Columbus to check out the cells in the spinal fluid and discuss options.

That did not happen. Richard agreed to be admitted to the hospital in Cleveland on December 16, to determine what was going on with himself. I decided to stay at the hospital but could not sleep well with the constant interruptions – better a well-rested princess than a grumpy one sleeping on a pea. Richard was experiencing fevers and extreme fatigue. Five days later my little energized bunny was discharged following hours of testing, infusion of antibiotics, anti-fungal drugs, bone marrow taps, neurological exams and audiology tests. He felt so much better that he abandoned his walker for one of many canes. This guy is a collector (part-time hoarder) of things he thinks he may need on any given day: knives, canes, pens, watches, colored pencils, gadgets, hats, reading glasses etc.

If anyone doubts the extent of the internal and external biome humans live with every day, observe Richard Hanson who has had close calls when the delicate balance between his immune system and the myriad bacteria, fungi, and viruses swirling in and out of him is disrupted.

On December 29, Richard sat enjoying a bowl of hot oatmeal, filled with raisins and brown sugar and reading the New York Times. Suddenly he began shaking, with chills and a reddish face. His temperature rose from 100.3 F. to 103.4 F within the hour. He made it to bed in a fleece jacket and hat and pulled the covers over his head. The doctor on call told me to take him to the emergency room, but I told her that I could not lift him or insure that he would not fall. "Call 911". Five 'burly men' came to 2425 and lifted him to the ambulance. In his confusion, Richard asked if they thought the Browns would win that day.

Yes, another infection with multiple "monster gram negative bugs' attacking this wonderful man had taken over and nestled in his port and back to his leg. His blood pressure dropped so low that I thought they might call a priest to administer last rites. Richard would probably agree to this despite his claim that he was an agnostic. He thought that he sometimes toyed with faith. The team pulled out their trusty toolbox and pumped him full of liquid soldiers to eradicate the foes.

Following the discharge on day 13, I observed that his physical needs had increased, and so I comply and carry his breakfast tray, warm his coffee and bring him his pills that we have carefully segregated according to time of day as I try to cope with this new level of care. Richard has been so self-reliant all of the years of our marriage, but now he needs more. Sometimes he calls out for me once too often, and I become easily irritated and impatient. I don't like this in myself and go into another room to utter some vulgar phrases, breathe deeply 3 times and tell myself that I can do this with kindness, courage and dedication.

Patience was never my strong suit, but I

certainly have cultivated this virtue lately so I don't run for the nearest exit. I lie to myself that this is only temporary. This too shall pass, and I will have my old Richard back as I trace my memories of the old days.

Richard has moved into the guest room where the height of the bed makes it easier for him to get up while holding onto his Rollator. This new arrangement is unfamiliar since we have been together in the same bed for most our 52.5-year marriage. The only other time we slept apart were 'those early morning Richard get-ups' to teach Biochemistry to the medical students or during those solo trips to deliver a talk at some university. It feels strange to give him his pills, put drops in his eyes, tuck him in, kiss him good night and close the door.

Gloria's Personal Blog

Another new arrangement is the preparation of three, albeit small, meals a day for him. He has been independent for breakfast and lunch so this is a small challenge and restricting. I don't want to leave him alone for very long, It took a while to adjust, but I am at peace with the new endgame phase of our lives.

It has been a demanding time since January 11, 2014 when Richard returned home from his long hospital stay with new antibiotics and antivirals for the cytomegalovirus making its home in his blood. He settled into his chair where he sits, reads and works on his computer. His hearing and energy levels are still problems, but we are working to find solutions like the 'Pocket Talker' that allows him to hear the TV without having the volume turned up enough to wake the dead. He eats the chicken soup provided by his personal chef, and his friends have been prohibited from talking of "checking out" but can utter positive thoughts to enhance the effects of the medications and chicken soup.

He is homebound except for trips to the doctors for treatment of his many ailments. These trips are challenges when snow and ice accumulate on the sidewalks, and I try to pry open doors and roll him to the patient Ford Fusion. My frequent gym workouts have been saving graces for my bones and my ability to push him around (in his transport chair, I mean). My gym rat friends are caring and supportive, filling my empty gas tank with encouragement and love. What would I do without them and family? I come home and fuss over my husband. We have established a routine where we snicker at Downton Abbey, laugh at Key and Peele and watch the Washington antics. Despairing thoughts are not allowed in our little bubble.

A ray of sunshine shone on Richard on January 30. Our grandson was walking to school past our condo in the morning. He usually waves, smiles and does a little dance shuffle. This morning, Hira was not smiling or waving. A few minutes later he buzzed asking to come upstairs. He 'fell' in and immediately covered his legs with a cover. He had underdressed for the frigid weather and was barely able to walk.

Following a hot cup of cocoa with whipped cream, he came alive and became his own charming self. He spent most of the day with us as he had no school to attend, but he did have a spelling list in preparation for a spelling bee. Grandpa took over the drills with his personalizing technique of using a word in a sentence involving Hira or his sports heroes. The mental activity tired the tutor so he went for a nap as his grandson walked with him to the bedroom and tucked him in. The visit was so therapeutic for Richard who relished spending time with the willing student, and was just as effective as the myriad pills he swallows each day.

Chapter 13

To Everything There is a Season

The news on February 6, 2014 was not what we wanted to hear. Richard's lungs harbor pneumonia and Respiratory Syncytial Virus, a common virus that can be easily controlled in healthy people, but that is not what we have here. We have a weakened fighter who can't fend off those numerous invaders, one who gets around with his Rollator, eats 3 mini-meals per day at the urging of the wife who has become the traditional Italian mamma who believes in the restorative power of food. I wish I had a robot to help me accomplish these caretaking chores, administer the antibiotics, flush the port, push him on his transport chair and help him into the car. Richard would not mind a mechanical helper – he would do anything to alleviate any stress on me.

How difficult to see my precious husband deteriorate before my very eyes. His arms are covered with large purple spots, pools of blood from his low platelets and poor blood exchange. He is a shadow of his former self with thin thighs, arms and legs. His body is no longer the meso-morphic sturdy male of yore, His face still brings forth his basic good looks, but his eyes don't sparkle as they used to do, and they have a faraway look as if he is following a spirit in his path. His voice is quiet, and his hearing minimal.

He is slipping away from me. I struggle to take care of him without taking away any fragment of independence he has left. This caretaking life is not so physically demanding, but it is restricting and emotionally draining. I feel a weariness and ennui that won't lift. I make myself go to the gym and exercise so I can sleep at night, but my heart is not in it. I see the older couples in the breakfast club and ask why we can't join them. I drift off and wonder what he is doing and shouldn't I be there with him. I long for peace, but that peace will come with a high price. I will lose my husband, my friend, my lover, and my life.

Why does it have to be this way?
Why couldn't we grow older together?
Why? Why? Why?"

Gloria's Personal Blog

There is a time to live.... Richard W. Hanson, my husband of 52 plus years, friend and confidante for 54 plus years, has decided on this 21st day of February to engage the hospice services at University Hospitals, who would keep him comfortable as he made his final journey. The quality of his life has been in decline for the past several months as he battles one infection after another with no help from his weakened immune system. He struggles to hear, walk and stay awake. Oxygen has become one of his best friends, allowing him to sit in the family room, work on manuscripts, write, take calls and watch the evening news with all of its horrors. He takes pleasure to watch Doc Martin with a little Laurence Welk beforehand as he reminisces about watching the bandleader with Bill and Dora, his beloved in-laws. No more do we giggle and poke fun at the fuddy-duddy show.

He responds to requests for visits from his friends and colleagues with sorrow and regret. He is too emotionally and physically exhausted. Only those few who persist are reluctantly invited to visit. During those times he digs deep inside that reservoir of energy to engage in short conversations – doing more listening than talking. He can communicate better with emails and short telephone conversation as he says good-bye.

Chapter 14

Finale - And So It Ends

At 8:15PM on February 28, 2014, Richard Winfield Hanson's body followed his blithesome spirit out of our world. Twenty years of struggle battling chronic lymphocytic leukemia, fifteen drugs to fight those mutated B cells, numerous clinical trials with new and promising drugs or combinations together with antibiotics, anti-fungals, anti-virals, blood product transfusions, oxygen, chicken soup, visits to every specialist imaginable, wondrous care by those oncology nurses. Love, affection and admiration kept him alive for those long years, albeit riding a roller coaster.

The costs in monetary terms for this battle were staggering: insurance costs and co-pays, travel expenses to and from Columbus, Ohio, hotel bills, food, medical supplies and special gadgets to keep him amused. Every penny spent was worth it since his struggles kept him alive for many years and will help others who wage the cancer battle. This altar boy, Eagle Scout, Army man, scientist, teacher, loyal husband, father and grandfather worked at his job until the last few weeks of his life and left a legacy of courage and determination.

He had been a supportive father figure for many young people who heard him lecture on the intricacies of metabolism and biochemistry and an inspiration to a generation of young scientists. His friends were a rare collection of individuals – both rich and poor, intellectually gifted and just plain Joes and Janes. He loved them all. He did not want to leave us – not any of us. Until the very end he was ready to fight on to defeat the infections and the cancer. That was not meant to be. He drifted off to another place where we will soon follow.

The mourning period never seems to end. It comes and goes, those retreats into the abyss of solitude, with its memories, forbidden desires and thoughts, alternating with hours and days filled with tablespoons of business. He left plenty for us to do to keep him alive in our memories, to keep us from the depths of despair.

Then there is the bewilderment, the dazed look and the claustrophobic feel of our home. There are so many things I miss: the spooning, the warm legs heating up my cold feet, the warm affectionate hugs and kisses, the grocery shopping relief, the singing, and hard to believe–the banjo playing.

I walk around among his things, doubting that he has gone forever. I move these items around and try to hide some so I can keep up the illusion that he will return and sort out his "stuff." The rest of my time is spent mending my broken heart as I go through the motions of being a widow and making attempts to re-fashion a new persona – not Mrs. Hanson or Mrs. Richard Hanson, but learning to say Gloria Hanson and accepting this new reality.

I calm myself with the thought that I was privileged to have had the opportunity to walk along side Richard as he fought the good fight with every tool available from modern science. We took advantage of any treatment that would prolong his life. These clinical trials were demanding, frustrating and ennobling for the patient and the caregiver, but even though the war was ultimately lost, the human spirit was the victor in this battle against these deadly diseases called cancer.

The following appendices have been added to give the reader a view of the scope and intensity of this fight for survival and relevance of a life.

CLINICAL TRIALS

Clinical trials for cancer are prospective studies designed to determine the safety of a drug in Phase 1 where the drug is given to a small number of patients and the doctors study the best way to deliver the drug and the proper dosage. In Phase 2 the researchers test the drug on a larger number of patients to determine if it works. In Phase 3 the drug is tested for efficacy in hundreds or thousands of patients. In this phase, the outcomes are compared to those receiving a placebo or a standard-of-care therapy. If a medication passes these 3 stages, approval for its use may be sought from the Food and drug administration.

Today more and more clinical trials are taking advantage of the diversity of the population in designing trials that target specific types of cancers. Patients are given excellent medical care when receiving the drugs and are carefully monitored as the trial progresses, after which, the statistical analysis of the results are made, and further determination is possible.

DRUGS TAKEN BY RICHARD FROM 1999-2114

Drug	year	remission
Fludarabine Cyclophosphomibe	2000	6 year
Dexamethasone Rituximab Fludaribine	2006	8 month
Bendamustine Rituximab	2008-10	8 month
Flavopiridol Lenalidomide	2011	3 month
Ibrutinib Ofatumumab	2011-12	17 months
EPOCH R (etoposide) (doxorubicin) (vincrastin) (cyclophosphamide) (rituvan)	2012	1 month
AR-42	2012	1 month

Cyclophosphamidie		
Rituximab	2012	2 month
Rituximab		
Dexamethasone	2013	2 month
Cytarabine		
Carfilzomib	2013	4 month
Rituximab		
Cladribine	2013	5 month

Tests Performed

Hundreds of blood draws
CT scans
PET scans
Magnetic Resonance Imaging MRI
Lumbar punctures
Neurological
Auditory

Note from Author: I found the following to be very helpful during this process.

Your Lab Results Decoded, by Holly St. Lifer,
AARP The Magazine, Feb. - March, 2012

Other Drugs for infections and symptoms:
Allopurinol
Amoxicillin
Bennadryl
CefTRIAXoneone
Ciprodex
Ethambutol
Flomax
Fluconazole
Fluticasone
Latanoprost
Leviquin
Lipitor
Lomotile
Lorazepam
Mupirocin
Neulasta
Neurontin
Nexium
Rifabutin
Sumlfamethoxazole (Bactrin)
Terazosin
Timilol
Tylenol
Valacyclovir
Valgancilovir
Voriconazole
Zithromax
Zolpidem

Medical Conditions Treated

Chronic Lymphocytic Leukemia
Anemia
Lymphadenopathy
Uveitis
Shingles
Tendinitis
Dyspepnia
Bronchiectasis
Baker's cyst
Broken radial head
Leptomeningeal metastases
Cervical degenerative Disc Disease
Ischemia in cranial nerve 3
Cervical stenosis in 4 and 5
Transaminitis
Ventricular arrhythmia
Urinary retention
Prostatitis
Bacterial infections
Viral infections
Protozoan infections
Toxoplasmosis
Torn meniscal tear
Broken ribs
Cellulitis